TALKS on HEALTH

LINCOLN S MIYASAKA

WESTBOW
PRESS
A DIVISION OF THOMAS NELSON

All the royalties of this book will be directed to charity.

WestBow Press books may be ordered through booksellers or by contacting:

WestBow Press
A Division of Thomas Nelson
1663 Liberty Drive
Bloomington, IN 47403
www.westbowpress.com
1 (866) 928-1240

ISBN: 978-1-4908-1425-4 (sc)
ISBN: 978-1-4908-1424-7 (e)

Library of Congress Control Number: 2013919846

Printed in the United States of America.

WestBow Press rev. date: 11/8/2013

Contents

Preface

You will welcome this book and want to read it carefully as soon as you can lay hands on it. Usually, doctors are too busy to write books, besides, why would they want to divulge secrets that are the source of their bread and butter?

I am very pleased with this book for many reasons. Dr. Lincoln Miyasaka is a practicing physician who is committed to preventive medicine as much as healing illness. Much more useful is the advice essential to living a healthy, fulfilled life than one in which one damages or destroys the only body you have and goes to a doctor for help in restoring it!

Dr. Lincoln is dedicated to giving really helpful advice, not only for the best possible care of the body, but of the mind and of the heart. After all, we humans are more than physical beings. Avoiding and curing anxiety and depression can be as important as curing a physical malady. Highly to be recommended is his quotation of scripture passages that are useful in fighting emotional sickness of all kinds. Indeed, the Bible has many principles that have presented solutions to a variety of problems and challenges that afflict the lives of many people.

This book brings valuable advice to those who suffer conflicts and doubts in their marriages. Love and respect are fundamental in a relationship between husband and wife, but many are at a loss as to how one can achieve them. Follow this book to discover the best way to reach you goals for a fulfilling marriage.

As for children, every parent wants well-behaved, loving children that honor their parents and uphold biblical values. Dr. Miyasaka presents valuable suggestions for raising children that will make their parents proud of them. In this day and time, more than ever before, family worship and church fellowship provide opportunities to lay foundations that will not crumble before the onslaughts of the media and education that are completely secular in outlook.

I was particularly grateful for the author's clear, strong stand for the true Christian faith. Jesus' question: "What good is it for a man to gain the whole world, yet forfeit his soul"? (Mk 8.36), is the kind of question that all doctors should ask. There can never be a serious doubt that a person's eternal destiny is far more important than living a healthy life, however good that may be.

So if you want my advice, read this book, take it to heart and pass it on.

To God be all the glory!
Russell Shedd, Ph.D.

Introduction

The World Health Organization defined that, "Health is a dynamic state of complete physical, mental, spiritual, and social well-being and not merely the absence of disease or infirmity."[1]

It is interesting that two thousand years before, Dr. Luke, a physician of the first century and author of two books in the Bible, described the growth of Jesus in these four areas: "Jesus grew in wisdom and stature, and in favor with God and men" (Luke 2:52).

Talks on Health is the result of encounters with my patients over the last five years as a family physician in Shanghai, as well as reflections in my own personal spiritual journey shared in our community. Its purpose is to provide some practical suggestions for a healthy life in these same four areas—physical, mental, social (family), and spiritual, in a Christian perspective—especially in a transcultural context.

---

[1] *Proposed Amendment to the Preamble of the Constitution of the World Health Organization as Contained In Resolution EB101.R2.* (Adopted at the 101st session of the executive board, eighth meeting, January 22, 1998.)

How to Stay Healthy

The other day a patient asked me, "How do physicians keep from getting sick since they see patients every day who are ill? Tell me the secret to staying healthy."

"Well," I said, "it isn't true that doctors never get sick. I usually get sick at least once or twice a year. What I do for myself and recommend for others is not a secret. Actually, it is simply common sense that we frequently forget."

Rest

When you move to a foreign country, you may get tired more easily. When you encounter a new culture, language, and environment, consider giving yourself one extra hour of sleep. If you sleep well, you can potentially avoid many health problems, such as stress, migraines, back pain, and common colds. Your immune system will take care of most of the germs you come in contact with. Take regular breaks at least once a week and longer breaks once or twice a year. If you are well rested, you will be more mentally and physically fit for work or school.

Exercise

Regular physical activity—walking, cycling, swimming, etc.—will reduce your risk of obesity, hypertension, diabetes, coronary artery disease, and high cholesterol. Exercise also helps to reduce stress and improve your self-esteem, sense of well-being, and general mood.

Healthy Diet

A great number of health problems come from an unhealthy diet. In most developed areas of the world, excessive amounts of high-caloric and processed food and outsized portions are problems. We need to eat a balanced diet that is low in fat and excess sugar while not forgetting vegetables and fruits, which are rich in vitamins and fiber.

Leisure

We need to work and study hard but also to relax, enjoy life, and spend time with family. One day a patient told me that he had been living in Shanghai for twenty years. I asked him what the biggest change in the city was during this period. He replied, "Speed of life. Before we didn't have as many options as we do today but we had more time to enjoy life—just walk in the park or have a cup of tea with your neighbor." Time should be a gift, not your taskmaster.

Make Friends

We all need to be part of a group. It can be family, friends, or a soccer team. This network will help support us when necessary. Everybody needs a group of friends to share their thoughts, feelings, and doubts with—someone who will just listen and stay with us no matter what happens. This group can support, encourage, and help each other.

Purpose of Life

We all need a purpose or goal in life; otherwise we may feel life is meaningless. Don't let time slip by. Find ways to use your gifts to serve others. There are many opportunities to serve the community in your city.

Avoid Dangerous Habits

Smoking—even passive smoking—increases your risk of cancer and coronary artery disease. Avoidance and cessation of tobacco use could potentially reduce the incidence and mortality from lung cancer by about 90 percent.

Alcohol consumption above recommended amounts is associated with multiple health problems, including motor vehicle crashes, suicide, violence, hypertension, mental health disorders, and alcohol dependence.

Unsafe sexual behavior risks not only include chlamydia, gonorrhea, HIV, syphilis, and HPV, but also intangibles such as shame, guilt, and depression, not only for the affected person but his or her family and friends. Avoid high-risk and inappropriate behavior.

Preventive Measures

Simple hygienic measures that will help keep you healthy include washing your hands frequently before eating and after using the toilet, as well as avoiding touching your eyes, nose, and mouth unless you have recently cleaned your hands.

Use seat belts whenever you travel in a car, a helmet when cycling, and protective gear when skating. Avoid tanning in salons, and apply sunscreen when you are out in the sun.

Keeping your vaccinations up to date is also critically important. Chicken pox, measles, mumps, polio, rubella, hepatitis A and B, diphtheria, pertussis, tetanus, meningitis, pneumonia, hemophilus, yellow fever, Japanese encephalitis, rabies, HPV, and influenza are diseases that caused death and suffering for innumerable people in the past but now can be prevented by vaccination. The HPV vaccination can also prevent cervical, other genital, and anal cancers, while the hepatitis B vaccine can prevent liver cancer.

Health Checkups

- Starting from birth, regular well-baby checkups are recommended to detect birth defects, follow growth and development, and update vaccinations.
- Periodic health maintenance visits are recommended every one to three years for adult patients under the age of fifty and annually for those who are older.
- The 2007 United States Preventive Services Task Force (USPSTF) guidelines advise screening every two years for people with SBP (systolic blood pressure, or the higher number of BP measurement) and DBP (diastolic blood pressure, or the lower number of BP measurement) below 120mmHg and 80mmHg, respectively, and yearly for persons with SBP 120 to 139mmHg or DBP 80 to 89mmHg.

- Women are recommended to have well-women checkups with pap smears starting at age twenty-one and pap smears plus an HPV screening at thirty years at least every three years.
- Breast cancer screenings (mammograms) are recommended for women between fifty and sixty-nine years old yearly. Women with a strong family history of breast and ovarian cancer should receive more-intensive screening.
- All males should discuss with their physicians screening for prostate cancer between the ages of fifty and sixty-nine
- Colon cancer screening is advised at age fifty and over for patients with an average risk for colorectal cancer and earlier for those with increased risk.
- Likewise, bone density scans are recommended between ages fifty and sixty-five with risk factors for osteoporosis (family history, smoking) and for all women over the age of sixty-five.
- Asking two simple questions about mood and anhedonia ("Over the past two weeks, have you felt down, depressed, or hopeless?" and "Over the past two weeks, have you felt little interest or pleasure in doing things?") can accurately detect people who should be further evaluated for depression.
- The American Diabetes Association (ADA) recommends screening for diabetes for patients age forty-five and older without risk factors. The ADA also recommends testing for diabetes in adults who are overweight or obese (BMI

≥25kg/m^2) and have one or more additional risk factors for diabetes.[2]

Lincoln Miyasaka, MD
Shanghai United Family Hospital & Clinics

[2]   www.uptodate.com/contents/overview-of-preventive-medicine-in-adults.

Anxiety: How to Avoid It

"Doctor, there is a forty-five-year-old man in room A with chest pain. Here's his ECG."

In the consultation room, I saw a tall, athletic, and well-dressed man who was breathing fast and sweating, with fear written all over his face. Heart rate and blood pressure were slightly elevated, but the rest of his physical exam and the ECG were normal. His complaints were chest pain, shortness of breath, and dizziness for the past hour. We needed to make sure he didn't have any life-threatening conditions, such as a heart attack, so blood tests were performed.

When I told him all the tests were normal, he seemed relieved and smiled.

He started explaining that he had been quite stressed recently. As the CEO of a multinational company, he was facing many difficult situations, constant international travel, and sleepless nights, and as a result, he was restless and tense. He continued to exercise occasionally, maintained a balanced diet and enjoyed a good family relationship, but something was just not right.

This was not the only patient I had with this complaint. I'd seen quite a few successful professionals and young people with the same symptoms, which was a sign that their bodies were trying to say something. Like a computer system that warns us when something is wrong, we are built with a similar feedback system to help keep us from danger and harm. It is like the body is saying, "Speed limit exceeded. Slow down. Wrong move."

These days life's speed has far exceeded its limits. In a world that thrives on immediacy, people are bombarded with constant requests for instant information twenty-four hours a day, 365 days a year. Even in the consultation room, patients are worried about their work and are constantly checking their mobile devices. They are physically there, but their minds are elsewhere. When they go on vacation to a remote area, if they find out there is no Internet connection, they feel uneasy and restless. What was meant to be leisure time turns into a tortured fear that something bad might happen while they are out of touch.

As there is day and night, we need time to engage and to disengage, time to work and to rest, time to connect and to disconnect. As there are spring, summer, autumn, and winter, there is time for productivity and growth but also a time for reclusion and restoration. Disregarding the laws and limits we were born with can lead to poor health.

The Japanese character for worry is 心配, which, broken into its two components, means: heart (心) distributed (配). A stressed person, worrying about thousands of things at the same time, has his or her heart and thoughts paralyzed and is consequently ineffective.

There are several types of anxiety, including:

1. Generalized anxiety disorder
2. Panic disorder

3. Social phobia
4. Specific phobia
5. Obsessive-compulsive disorder
6. Acute stress disorder
7. Post-traumatic stress disorder

Symptoms and signs of anxiety may include:

1. Restlessness
2. Sweating
3. Palpitation, high blood pressure
4. Tingling
5. Dizziness, fainting, and headaches
6. Cold hands and feet
7. Dry mouth
8. Diarrhea, stomach pain
9. Insomnia

If you have any of these symptoms, my recommendation is for you to listen to these warnings. Stop and take time to analyze your life. Thoroughly check all your hardware and software—heart and mind, thoughts and feelings—and then follow these simple instructions:

1. Identify each problem. Write down everything that is not right.
2. Identify potential solutions. What are your options? Write down what needs to be done.

3. Fix the problems. Do what must be done, but focus on one thing at a time.

Finally, remember that exercise and a balanced diet are very important, as well as getting enough rest and sleep. The added daily stress of living in a foreign country means expatriates should be getting an additional hour of rest per day. Perhaps most importantly, a supportive network of family and friends is essential for a healthy life. Lastly, if your anxiety and stress continues to overwhelm you and negatively affect your life, please seek professional help.

Lincoln Miyasaka, MD
Shanghai United Family Hospital & Clinics

Inspirational Verses

Therefore I tell you, do not worry about your life, what you will eat or drink; or about your body, what you will wear. Is not life more than food, and the body more than clothes? Look at the birds of the air; they do not sow or reap or store away in barns, and yet your heavenly Father feeds them. Are you not much more valuable than they? Can any one of you by worrying add a single hour to your life? And why do you worry about clothes? See how the flowers of the field grow. They do not labor or spin. Yet I tell you that not even Solomon in all his splendor was dressed like one of these. If that is how God clothes the grass of the field, which is here today and tomorrow is thrown into the fire, will he not much more clothe you—you of little faith? So do not worry, saying, 'What shall we eat?' or 'What shall we drink?' or 'What shall we wear?' For the pagans run after all these things, and your heavenly Father knows that you need them. But seek first his kingdom and his righteousness, and all these things will be given to you as well. Therefore do not worry about tomorrow, for tomorrow will worry about itself. Each day has enough trouble of its own. (Matt. 6:25–34 NIV)

Question: What is the relationship between anxiety and faith according to the text?

Rejoice in the Lord always. I will say it again: Rejoice! Let your gentleness be evident to all. The Lord is near. Do not be anxious about anything, but in every situation, by prayer and petition, with thanksgiving, present your requests to God. And the peace of God, which transcends all understanding, will guard your hearts and your minds in Christ Jesus. Finally, brothers and sisters, whatever is true, whatever is noble, whatever is right, whatever is pure, whatever is lovely, whatever is admirable—if anything is excellent or praiseworthy—think about such things. Whatever you have learned or received or heard from me, or seen in me—put it into practice. And the God of peace will be with you. (Phil. 4:4–9 NIV)

Question: According to Paul, what do we need to do when we have a problem?

What kind of thoughts should we allow in our minds?

Recommended reading: David H. Barlow and Michelle Craske, *Mastery of Your Anxiety and Panic.* Oxford, UK: Oxford University Press, 2007.

Depression

Many years ago, I saw a thirty-year-old patient who came to the hospital with her mother and young daughter complaining of stomach pains. The physical examination was normal, but I noted she was very quiet the entire time. I was about to prescribe medication for her stomach when the mother spoke up, informing me that the patient had lost twelve kilograms within the last year, and after the birth of the patient's daughter, the patient's husband had begun to drink heavily and abuse her nearly every day. She was not eating or sleeping, cried all the time, and even admitted to suicidal thoughts. Therefore, instead of leaving with a medication for gastritis, I admitted my patient for treatment of severe depression. The lesson I learned from her is the critical importance of observation while simultaneously being available and making the time to give patients the opportunity to talk and ask questions. These lessons can also apply in relation to our friends and family members.

In stressful environments like Shanghai, we may at times feel tired and overburdened, have a lack of energy and motivation, or even feel worthless and hopeless. If these symptoms are mild and don't affect your daily life, they may be transitory, but if they are impacting your work, school grades, or family relationships, then it is wise to ask for professional advice and help.

Depression is a whole-person disorder that includes biological, psychological, and social aspects, but the fortunate news is there are effective treatments available. According to studies, four to five percent of the population suffers from some form of depression, while 17 percent have had or will have depression at some stage in their life. Between 10 and 14 percent of patients visiting a primary care physician have depression, but unfortunately only one-third of sufferers ever receive appropriate diagnosis and treatment.

Symptoms of depression include:

- depressed mood
- diminished interest or pleasure
- weight loss or gain
- insomnia or hypersomnia
- agitation
- fatigue or loss of energy
- feelings of uselessness and worthlessness or excessive or inappropriate guilt
- indecisiveness or decreased reasoning ability and concentration
- recurrent thoughts of death or suicide

Depression can be caused by biological and genetic factors. In addition, environmental factors, such as the death of someone close, separation or divorce, changes in employment—including a promotion—can lead to depression. Overwork, a lack of rest, failures on exams or at work, rejection, or any situation that ends in frustration and guilt are all other common catalysts. The consequences of untreated depression can be enormous, often resulting in personal and family suffering, professional regression, alcohol or other substance abuse, increased risk of accidents, or suicide.

Successful treatment of depression often includes a combination of therapy, medication, and rest. However, the first and arguably most important steps in treatment are to recognize you are depressed and seek treatment from a qualified healthcare professional. If any of what I have said sounds like I am describing you or someone close to you, I encourage you to talk to your family doctor or mental health specialist immediately.

Lincoln Miyasaka, MD
Shanghai United Family Hospital & Clinics

References

Diagnostic and Statistical Manual of Mental Disorders. Fourth Edition. Revision (DSM-IV-TR). American Psychiatric Association, 2000.

Leon AC, et al. "Prevalence of Mental Disorders in Primary Care: Implications for Screening." *Archives of Family Medicine.* 1995; 4(10): 857–61.

Maurer, DM. "Screening for Depression." *American Family Physician.* January 15, 2012; 85(2).

Sharp, LK and Lipsky, MS. "Screening for Depression across the Lifespan: A Review of Measures for Use in Primary Care Settings." American Family Physician. September 15, 2002; 66(6):1001–9.

David B. Biebel and Harold G. Koenig, *New Light on Depression.* Grand Rapids, MI: Zondervan, 2010.

Inspirational Verses

Lessons from David

In the spring, at the time when kings go off to war, David sent Joab out with the king's men and the whole Israelite army. They destroyed the Ammonites and besieged Rabbah. But David remained in Jerusalem. One evening David got up from his bed and walked around on the roof of the palace. From the roof he saw a woman bathing. The woman was very beautiful, and David sent someone to find out about her. The man said, "She is Bathsheba, the daughter of Eliam and the wife of Uriah the Hittite." Then David sent messengers to get her. She came to him, and he slept with her. (2 Sam. 11:1–4)

For the director of music. A psalm of David. When the prophet Nathan came to him after David had committed adultery with Bathsheba.

Have mercy on me, O God, according to your unfailing love; according to your great compassion blot out my transgressions. Wash away all my iniquity and cleanse me from my sin. For I know my transgressions, and my sin is always before me. Against you, you only, have I sinned and done what is evil in your sight; so you are right in your verdict and justified when you judge. Surely I was sinful at birth, sinful from the time my mother conceived me. Yet you desired faithfulness even in the womb; you taught me wisdom in that secret place. Cleanse me with hyssop, and I will be clean; wash me, and I will be whiter than snow. Let me hear joy and gladness; let the bones you have crushed rejoice. Hide your face from my sins and blot out all my iniquity. Create in me a pure heart, O God, and renew a steadfast spirit within me. (Ps. 51:1–10 NIV)

Blessed is the one whose transgressions are forgiven, whose sins are covered. Blessed is the one whose sin the Lord does not count against them and in whose spirit is no deceit. When I kept silent, my bones wasted away through my groaning all day long. For day and night your hand was heavy on me; my strength was sapped as in the heat of summer. Then I acknowledged my sin to you and did not cover up my iniquity. I said, "I will confess my transgressions to the Lord." And you forgave the guilt of my sin. (Ps. 32:1–5)

Do you recognize symptoms of depression in these texts?

What happens when we break the law or our code of ethics?

What did David do to solve his problem, and what was the result?

Lessons from Solomon

"Meaningless! Meaningless!" says the Teacher. "Utterly meaningless! Everything is meaningless. What do people gain from all their labors at which they toil under the sun?" (Eccles. 1:2–3)

I, the Teacher, was king over Israel in Jerusalem. I applied my mind to study and to explore by wisdom all that is done under the heavens. What a heavy burden God has laid on mankind! I have seen all the things that are done under the sun; all of them are meaningless, a chasing after the wind. (Eccles. 1:12–14)

I said to myself, "Look, I have increased in wisdom more than anyone who has ruled over Jerusalem before me; I have experienced much of wisdom and knowledge." Then I applied myself to the understanding of wisdom, and also of madness and folly, but I learned that this, too, is a chasing after the wind. (Eccles. 1:16–17)

Yet when I surveyed all that my hands had done and what I had toiled to achieve, everything was meaningless, a chasing after the wind; nothing was gained under the sun. (Eccles. 2:11)

> So I hated life, because the work that is done under the sun was grievous to me. All of it is meaningless, a chasing after the wind. (Eccles. 2:17)

> Remember your Creator in the days of your youth, before the days of trouble come and the years approach when you will say, "I find no pleasure in them." (Eccles. 12:1)

All humans have deep inside a cry for love, for security, and for significance. There is an existential emptiness that nothing in this world can fill because this hole is the size of God.

Lessons from Elijah

> Now Ahab told Jezebel everything Elijah had done and how he had killed all the prophets with the sword. So Jezebel sent a messenger to Elijah to say, "May the gods deal with me, be it ever so severely, if by this time tomorrow I do not make your life like that of one of them." Elijah was afraid and ran for his life. When he came to Beersheba in Judah, he left his servant there, while he himself went a day's journey into the wilderness. He came to a broom bush, sat down under it and prayed that he might die. "I have had enough, Lord," he said. "Take my life; I am no better than my ancestors." Then he lay down under the bush and fell asleep. All at once an angel touched him and said, "Get up and eat." He looked around, and there by his head was some bread baked over hot coals, and a jar of water. He ate and drank and then lay down

again. The angel of the Lord came back a second time and touched him and said, "Get up and eat, for the journey is too much for you." So he got up and ate and drank. Strengthened by that food, he traveled forty days and forty nights until he reached Horeb, the mountain of God. There he went into a cave and spent the night. And the word of the Lord came to him: "What are you doing here, Elijah?" He replied, "I have been very zealous for the Lord God Almighty. The Israelites have rejected your covenant, torn down your altars, and put your prophets to death with the sword. I am the only one left, and now they are trying to kill me too." The Lord said, "Go out and stand on the mountain in the presence of the Lord, for the Lord is about to pass by." Then a great and powerful wind tore the mountains apart and shattered the rocks before the Lord, but the Lord was not in the wind. After the wind there was an earthquake, but the Lord was not in the earthquake. After the earthquake came a fire, but the Lord was not in the fire. And after the fire came a gentle whisper. When Elijah heard it, he pulled his cloak over his face and went out and stood at the mouth of the cave. (1 Kings 19:1–13)

Elijah was a faithful servant of God, preaching His Word fearlessly in an ungodly society. He was persecuted and felt alone and exhausted. He even wanted to die. Did God rebuke him? No, He allowed him to rest, gave him food, and showed that He was there for him.

Family

Parents today have very long workdays and almost no contact with their children and with each other. A patient who was going through a divorce told me, "I used to be a powerful man a few years ago, proud, rich, important, but now I have lost my job, my family, and my health. I have nothing." Certainly we need to work, but what is the purpose of it if we lose our families? Family is so important to our emotional health, sense of well-being, and happiness.

Children who do not receive affection and love as they grow develop mistrust of people, insecurity, and low self-image. Dr. Loren Moshen of the National Institute of Mental Health, which analyzed the national census figures, found that a father's absence is a more prominent factor than poverty in juvenile delinquency. A study of thirty-nine adolescent girls suffering from anorexia nervosa showed that thirty-six of them had one common denominator: a lack of a good relationship with their fathers [3].

Today's society is controlled by the media.

The media is constantly bombarding the minds of our children with scenes of violence and sex. The lessons they are instilling is

---

[3]   Josh McDowell and Dr Norm Wakefield, The Dad Difference, USA, Here's Life Publishers, 1989

that the hero is no longer the one who does good deeds but who tricks and cheats others. The values of today's society are reversed.

There is a tendency in society not to restrain children, to leave them free to develop their potential. That is why many parents today raise their children as visitors, like little kings in their homes, creating in them the characteristics of impulsiveness and inability to repress desires. Today's children have a higher level of antisocial behavior than the previous generation [4].

Children have very few adult friends. The group's influence is very strong. Many times children do not want to do certain things, but as everyone does, they end up doing them. It is said that the youth and adolescents of different nations have more in common than parents and children from the same families because there is little or no significant relationship between parents and their children. Children are required to grow up too fast. They are exposed to adult themes early in life. Even children's programs are permeated with sensuality. We live in a hedonistic society (that values pleasure) with a low level of morality.

We need to have a critical view so we are not washed away in the flow of this world. The best we can do is read what God, our Creator, recommends about family and marriage. In the Bible, the owner's manual for life, we find some wise advice: "Do not conform to the pattern of this world, but be transformed by the renewing of your mind. Then you will be able to test and approve what God's will is—his good, pleasing and perfect will" (Rom. 12:2).

---

[4]   Josh McDowell and Dr Norm Wakefield, The Dad Difference, USA, Here's Life Publishers, 1989

God's Principles for Dating

People's future spouses will be chosen during the dating stage, so we can say that dating begins the foundation of the future family. The liberal teachings transmitted by the media and society today concerning dating, as well as novels and films, are very questionable. They do not show the bitterness, guilt, shame, fear, diseases, unplanned pregnancies, and even death that can result—the sad end of a "liberated life."

In Genesis 1:27, we read about the creation of sex. Sex is wonderful. It is blessed by God but only within marriage (Gen. 2:18–25). One young man asked his father, "What is safe sex?" The father replied, "A wedding ring on your finger!" Sex is 100 percent safe only when both partners are faithful in marriage. The Bible says the fear of the Lord is the beginning of wisdom. The young would be wise to replace bad thoughts with good habits, study, work, sports, and good reading. "How can a young person stay on the path of purity? By living according to your word" (Ps. 119:9).

Instructions for Marriage in Genesis 2:18–25

> The Lord God said, "It is not good for the man to be alone. I will make a helper suitable for him." Now the Lord God had formed out of the ground all the wild animals and all the birds in the sky. He brought them to the man to see what he would name them; and whatever the man called each living creature, that was its name. So the man gave names to all the livestock, the birds in the sky and all the wild animals. But for

Adam no suitable helper was found. So the Lord God caused the man to fall into a deep sleep; and while he was sleeping, he took one of the man's ribs and then closed up the place with flesh. Then the Lord God made a woman from the rib he had taken out of the man, and he brought her to the man. The man said, "This is now bone of my bones and flesh of my flesh; she shall be called 'woman,' for she was taken out of man." That is why a man leaves his father and mother and is united to his wife, and they become one flesh. Adam and his wife were both naked, and they felt no shame.

1. "A man leaves his father and mother …"

The union of a man and a woman cannot be ephemeral, uncompromising, "hanging" for a while, or until they find a more interesting relationship. There is a milestone, a change in marital status from single to married. You are not single anymore. The old things are past, and many things you did as a single person would not be appropriate now. You cannot just spend all day playing soccer with your friends as you used to. Emotionally there should also be a change or a cut in the umbilical cord. You cannot compare your wife with your mother or your husband with your father. "She does not even know how to cook. Why she does not as my mother does?"

For parents we see the fulfillment of the mission of motherhood and fatherhood. Parents need to know that although they continue to be fathers and mothers, they have fulfilled their responsibility to raise their children. Thus parents should release their children to follow their lives, starting in their own homes. Marriage means to leave your original core family to set up a new family. Now the responsibility in the new home is with the newlywed couple and no one else.

2. "United to his wife ..."

Marriage is a union. It's like gluing two sheets of paper together. You cannot separate without ripping them apart. Mark 10:6–12 says: "Therefore what God has joined together, let no one separate." Alliance or covenant in Hebrew is *berith*. It involves two elements: love (*ahab*) and faithfulness, loyalty (*chesed*) [5]. Marriage is a commitment of love and faithfulness, unalterable and permanent bond in nature. Many people confuse love with passion. Passion is a temporary feeling and an unstable emotion. First Corinthians 13:1–9 tells us what love is.

> If I speak in the tongues of men or of angels, but do not have love, I am only a resounding gong or a clanging cymbal. If I have the gift of prophecy and can fathom all mysteries and all knowledge, and if I have a faith that can move mountains, but do not have love, I am nothing. If I give all I possess to the poor and give over my body to hardship that I may boast, but do not have love, I gain nothing. Love is patient, love is kind. It does not envy, it does not boast, it is not proud. It does not dishonor others, it is not

---

[5] W.E. Vine, An Expository Dictionary of Biblical Words, Thomas Nelson Publishers, Nashville, TN, 1984; E.F.Harrison, Baker's Dictionary of Theology, Baker Book House, Grand Rapids, MI, 1960

self-seeking, it is not easily angered, it keeps no record of wrongs. Love does not delight in evil but rejoices with the truth. It always protects, always trusts, always hopes, always perseveres. Love never fails.

3. "And they become one flesh …"

Marriage is the most intimate relationship between two people, but it is a process. It requires time. Cultivating a relationship is like cultivating a garden or a flower. It takes patience, perseverance, communication, forgiveness, and adaptation. For this union to happen, we cannot think, *How can I change him or her?* Instead we must ask God what needs to be changed in me. How can we be better husbands or better wives? Brokenness and mutual submission are the ingredients to became one flesh. Have you seen some couples who have been together for forty or fifty years? They have faced many problems together and walked together for so long that they seem like siblings. The other day I was walking in front of the hospital and stopped to see an old couple. A very thin husband was holding his wife's hand and helping her go up the stairs. What a lovely scene! You must become one flesh.

4. "They were both naked, and they felt no shame" (Gen. 2:25). The man and woman were pure—naked physically but covered by the glory of God. They had no barriers between God and between each other. Transparency. Intimacy. Communion. Friendship. We need to talk and communicate clearly and lovingly all the time.

The Role of the Husband

Love your wife. In Ephesians 5:25–33 it is written four times, "Love your wife" as Christ loved the church. Christ loved the church so much that He gave His life for her. If the husband does not love his wife as Christ loved His church, he is disobeying God.

True love is not conditional to the behavior, appearance, or attitude of the beloved. Hosea was a prophet whose wife left home and gave herself to prostitution. He went after her for love. He found her being sold into slavery. He paid the price and restored her as his wife. This is a picture of what Christ did for us. While we were unfaithful to Him, He came after us and paid with His own life to rescue and restore us. This kind of love is a result of our relationship with God. "But the fruit of the Spirit is love, joy, peace, forbearance, kindness, goodness, faithfulness, gentleness and self-control. Against such things there is no law" (Gal. 5:22–23).

The Role of the Wife

> Wives, submit yourselves to your own husbands as you do to the Lord. For the husband is the head of the wife as Christ is the head of the church, his body, of which he is the Savior. Now as the church submits to Christ, so also wives should submit to their husbands in everything … and the wife must respect her husband. (Eph. 5:22–24, 33b).

Often to "be submissive" sounds like something that is too outdated for our modern society, where women have earned their space, their rights, and equality before men. Or maybe it seems like something negative and humiliating.

However, this passage speaks of the respect and honor she should treat her husband with. It means careful consideration in words and attitudes. In a lecture on marriage, a counselor commented on the thousands of books that address the topic. There are countless theories and advice, but he said, actually it is very simple: husband, love your wife, and wife, respect your husband. The Word of God is clear and objective. God knows what a woman needs: to be loved. Also He knows what the man needs: to be respected, especially by his mate. And because He knows it is difficult and sometimes an almost impossible task for the couple, He leaves these commands recorded in a clear and even repetitive way. But a woman who is truly loved naturally corresponds with respect to her husband. Likewise, the man who is respected and valued loves more intensely. Love includes respect, and respect reveals love. It is submission to one another.

Children

> Children, obey your parents in the Lord, for this is right. "Honor your father and mother"—which is the first commandment with a promise—"so that it may go well with you and that you may enjoy long life on the earth." Honor thy father and thy mother. (Eph. 6:1–4)

To honor means obeying with love. "Obey" is a commandment. If you are not honoring your parents, you are disobeying God. This commandment has a promise attached to it: "So that it may

go well with you and that you may enjoy long life on the earth."
Oyakouko is a Japanese word that means respectful love. That is
typical of Asian culture, and we want to preserve it.

Parents

"Fathers, do not exasperate your children; instead, bring them up
in the training and instruction of the Lord."

1. Discipline. Set limits.

When you say yes, yes it is, and when you say no, it is no. A certain
mother saw her son doing something she considered wrong and
told him to stop. The son continued as if he heard nothing. His
mother repeated the order, and he continued to do the action. The
mother began to get nervous and increased the tone of her voice.
She came to the point where she lost control, lifted the child up,
and threw him to the ground. It all started because she did not
make her words count. We must teach obedience and respect,
and that will be invaluable throughout your children's life. Start
early, preferably from birth. The first three to four years are the
most important. At this young age, children need to be taught
obedience and limits for their own good. Discipline and limits are
essential. However, we must emphasize that in no way can it be
done in anger or violence, but it should be an expression of love
so the child understands why she is being disciplined.

> No discipline seems pleasant at the time, but
> painful. Later on, however, it produces a harvest of
> righteousness and peace for those who have been
> trained by it. (Heb. 12:11)

A rod and a reprimand impart wisdom, but a child left undisciplined disgraces its mother. (Prov. 29:15)

Discipline your children, and they will give you peace; they will bring you the delights you desire. (Prov. 29:17)

Those whom I love I rebuke and discipline. So be earnest and repent. (Rev. 3:19)

2. Cultivate a relationship.
   a. Be present. Be available. Make plans with your children, talk, and take time with each child.
   b. Be transparent. Recognize your mistakes.
   c. Respect him or her as a person. Some parents try to fulfill in their children their own dreams, expecting them to be what they couldn't. Instead, respect your child's life and will.
   d. Encourage. Keep the ratio of four times more recognition (praise) for every rebuke.

3. Love the mother of your children.
Patrick Makergot, an English missionary who has been in Japan since 1965, said the best thing you can do for your child is to love his mother.

In his book *The Total Man*, Dan Benson reports the value of the moments of childhood.

I will never forget the hugs in family that always took place in our kitchen when I was growing. Crawling

31

through the door I saw mommy involved in daddy's arms (this was not an unusual scene in our house). It made me feel good inside. So well that I could not resist and joined myself to them. I went around the room that led me to where they were and grabbed his legs. Mom and Dad were always happy to include me. If some of the other brothers were around, they sometimes joined us, and the family's embrace grew larger and larger. Mom and Dad made our house a loving home, more by example than by lecturing. We had safety as children because Daddy took the lead and the atmosphere in our home was of love and joy[6].

4. Be an example.

Dennis Rainey in his book *Pulling Weeds, Planting Seeds* devoted two entire chapters as a tribute to his mother and his father. He says,

> As a sensitive child, my radar picked up much of the life of my father than he imagined. During the dangerous years of adolescence, he was the model and hero I needed—and still is. He taught me the importance of hard work and complete a task. I learned about the long-term commitment with him— never feared my parents got divorced. My father was absolutely dedicated to my mother. I felt safe and protected. More importantly, he taught me about the character. He did what was right, even when no one was looking. Never heard about not paying

---

6   Dan Benson, *The Total Man*, Tyndale house Pub, 1977

taxes—he paid without grumbling. His integrity was impeccable. I never heard him lie and his eyes always demanded the same truth in return. The mental image of his character still fuels and energizes my life today[7].

5. Have family worship.

> Hear, O Israel: The Lord our God, the Lord is one. Love the Lord your God with all your heart and with all your soul and with all your strength. These commandments that I give you today are to be on your hearts. Impress them on your children. Talk about them when you sit at home and when you walk along the road, when you lie down and when you get up. (Deut. 6:4–7)

Children are precious gifts granted by God that we were given the honor to love, to take care of for a while, and to try to be a good example with the prayer that one day they will be able to know the Lord and follow him.

Recommended Books

1. J.C. of Ferrières, Purer than diamond, Scripture Union Press & Books. (2010)
2. J. Kemp, Eu amo você namoro, noivado, casamento e sexo, United Press 2005
3. F. Lawes, S. Olford The Sanctity of Sex,. Fleming H Revell Co, [Westwood, N.J.], 1963

Dennis Rainey, *Pulling Weeds, Planting Seeds*. Here's Life Publisher, 1989

4. L. Palau, Con Quien Me Casare? Whom shall I Marry, Editorial Unilit, 2011

5. R. E. Short, Sex, Love or Romance, Fell, Frederick Publishers, Incorporated, 2003

6. W. Trobisch, Love is a Feeling to Be Learned, Quiet Waters Publications, 2009

7. J. McDowell, Teens Speak Out, USA, Here's Life Publishers, 1987

8. J. McDowell and Dr Norm Wakefield, The Dad Difference, USA, Here's Life Publishers, 1989

9. J. M. Drescher, When your child is 6 -12, Herald Press, 198610.

10. W. F. Harley, Jr, His Needs Her Needs, Fleming H Revell, Grand Rapids, 2001

Spirituality and Health

Faith reduces the rate of suicide, depression, and anxiety and improves quality of life of patients.[8]

Religious involvement is associated with:

- greater well-being and happiness;
- less depression and faster recovery from depression;
- significantly greater meaning and purpose in life;
- significantly greater hope;
- significantly more forgiveness;
- significantly more altruism/volunteering; and
- significantly more gratitude[9].

THE ONE THING

The LORD is my light and my salvation—whom shall I fear? The LORD is the stronghold of my life—of whom shall I be afraid? When the wicked advance against me to devour me, it is my enemies and my foes who will stumble and fall. Though an army besiege me, my heart will not fear; though war break out

---

[8] Harold G. Koenig, geriatrician and psychiatrist of Duke University

[9] Handbook of Religion and Health, Systematic Review, Harold G. Koenig, Michael E. McCullough, David B. Larson. (Oxford, UK: Oxford University Press, 2001).

> against me, even then I will be confident. One thing
> I ask from the LORD, this only do I seek: that I may
> dwell in the house of the LORD all the days of my
> life, to gaze on the beauty of the LORD and to seek
> him in his temple. (Ps. 27:1–4)

John Calvin (1509–1564), the influential French theologian, used to say that the book of Psalms is

> "an Anatomy of all the Parts of the Soul;" for there
> is not an emotion of which any one can be conscious
> that is not here represented as in a mirror. The Holy
> Spirit has drawn to the life all the grieves, sorrows,
> fears, doubts, hopes, cares, perplexities, in short, all
> the distracting emotions with which the minds of men
> are wont to be agitated. [10]

He is saying that in the Psalms, we can see as in a mirror reflected faithfully all the emotions of the human soul. Psalms is one of the most cherished books ever written because it talks from the heart about heart issues of real-life experience with all its struggles and complications.

Although today humanity is subject to all kinds of emotional afflictions, there was a time when man was completely free of concerns, worries, and fears. He had complete joy and perfect love, walked in holiness, and enjoyed wonderful and perfect peace with God, with himself, with other humans, and with nature. Then one day he disobeyed God, as is described in Genesis 3:

---

[10]   www.studylight.org/com/cal

Then the man and his wife heard the sound of the
Lord God as he was walking in the garden in the cool
of the day, and they hid from the Lord God among
the trees of the garden. But the Lord God called to the
man, "Where are you?" He answered, "I heard you in
the garden, and I was afraid because I was naked; so
I hid." (Gen. 3:8–10)

The first couple knew they had sinned against God and
experienced fear and shame for the first time in their lives. This
fear passed to all generations after them, as we can see throughout
human history till this day.

According to Kessler, the lifetime prevalence of anxiety is
28.8 percent of the adult population in the United States, and the
average age of onset is eleven years old.[11] Nowadays anxiety, worry,
fear, stress, and restlessness are very common in any culture, in
any place, in any age.

There are places in this world where war, armies, and bombings
are a daily menace to people's lives, as we can see in the news
almost every day. Fortunately, we don't have this problem right
now in this country, but certainly there are other types of battles
and struggles in our modern lives that make us anxious as well.

Time is a gift from God, but the world system has turned
it into our taskmaster, increasing the speed of life and making
the goal for many people today just productivity, growth, and

---

[11]   Kessler RC, Berglund PA, Demler O, Jin R, Walters EE. Lifetime
prevalence and age-of-onset distributions of DSM-IV disorders in the
National Comorbidity Survey Replication (NCS-R). *Archives of General
Psychiatry.* 2005 Jun; 62(6): 593–602.

competition. People all over the world keep running all the time, working fifteen to seventeen hours a day, seven days a week. They are so high speed that they cannot slow down, turn off their minds, or sleep anymore. Try to drive a car over 140 km/h all the time. Observe what happens in your body: you get tense, your heart beats fast, your pupils are dilated, and your whole system gets prepared for danger so it can react quickly to any menace that might happen. This is what happens if the speed in your life is above the limit you were designed for.

Because of the high speed in life, people tend to do many things at the same time. They will read a book, listen to music, send e-mail, and talk on the phone all at the same time in this multitasking generation. When they are walking, they are physically there, but their thoughts are completely in another realm. I see many patients, especially male patients, who come to the office, but their minds and hearts are elsewhere. They are constantly looking the iPhone, iPad, iSomething. They say, "I am sorry, but I need to reply to this." When they go on vacation and find out that there is no Internet access, they start to feel uneasy and breathless, and they will panic if they are not able to connect with the world. What was meant to be a relaxing vacation turns out to be a traumatic event because they feel like something terrible will happen. We need to remember that we are still humans. We need to respect our limits. We need rest, exercise, and family time. We need to engage but also to disengage, to work but also to rest.

Another characteristic of our times is that there are too many options to choose. There are so many shopping centers with so many products and so many things to do that we get lost. I remember Prof. Russell Shedd, one of the most-respected Bible teachers in Brazil, talking about his father, a missionary in Bolivia, when he went back to United States and entered a shopping center by the first time. He said, "I never saw a place with so many things together that I don't need." All these things and options bring not only an emptiness to our hearts (because none of these things can fill the hole inside of us) but also make us anxious, stressed, nervous, tense, uneasy, and restless.

David shared a way he found to overcome fear and anxiety in his life. He said, "The Lord is my light and my salvation—whom shall I fear? The Lord is the stronghold of my life—of whom shall I be afraid?" David was an unusual man, inspired poet, gifted musician, and great soldier and leader. He was the best king of Israel ever, but what was his purpose in life? Wealth? Power? Position? To be the king? No, all these things were quite incidental. He said, "One thing have I desired of the Lord, that will I seek after." He had just one thing, one purpose, one desire, and one goal only. He not only wanted and desired it, but he sought after it. His passion, purpose, and one goal in life, as he said, was, "To dwell in the house of the Lord all the days of my life." To dwell is to be there, to live there, and to remain there. Our dwelling is our home, our base, where we are comfortable. It is where we come back to every day from wherever we go, where we abide. David's one desire was to be with the Lord, to stay in His presence, to walk with Him, and to sit at His feet all the days of his life. In the Lord's presence David found rest, shelter, and comfort. He found a dwelling place, a refuge in the house of the Lord.

David's life was never easy. Even as a young shepherd, he was attacked by a lion and a bear. He had wicked people around him and enemies and foes trying to eat up his flesh. There was hosts encamping around him and war rising against him. Do you remember when Goliath came to challenge Israel?

> His height was six cubits and a span (about nine feet nine inches or three meters high). He had a bronze helmet on his head and wore a coat of scale armor of bronze weighing five thousand shekels (about 125 pounds or fifty-eight kilograms); on his legs he wore bronze greaves, and a bronze javelin was slung on his back. His spear shaft was like a weaver's rod, and its iron point weighed six hundred shekels (fifteen pounds or about 6.9 kilograms) I Samuel 17:4-7

It would be natural to feel afraid, worried, or panicked facing a giant like that, but David, even as a young boy, was confident. Why? He said, "The Lord who rescued me from the paw of the lion and the paw of the bear will rescue me from the hand of this Philistine." And he said to Goliath, "You come against me with sword and spear and javelin, but I come against you in the name of the Lord Almighty, the God of the armies of Israel, whom you have defied" (1 Samuel 17).

David was confident because his audience was not the armies of the Philistines or Goliath. His audience was the Lord God almighty, in whose presence he was dwelling. Before the greatness of his Lord, all his enemies looked like tiny, harmless pygmies. Are you facing some giants today? Are you worried about a situation you cannot handle? Dwell in the house of the Lord, and you will find rest and refuge in His presence. David told us two reasons why he wanted to dwell in the house of the Lord. One was to behold the beauty of the Lord—to admire, to gaze, to contemplate, and to let all the cells of his brain be impressed by His beauty, glory, and holiness. He also desired to bow down before the majesty, immensity, and greatness of his Lord—to praise and exalt Him forever.

The temple, the house of the Lord, was a place of worship and David's one desire, one goal, and one purpose was to be with the Lord all the days of his life, to behold His beauty and worship Him.

One of the most influential Christian thinkers and writers of the last century was C. S. Lewis, author of *The Chronicles of Narnia* and professor at Oxford University (1898–1963). He said,

> When I first began to draw near to belief in God and even for some time after it had been given to me, I found a stumbling block in the demand so clamorously made by all religious people that we should "praise" God; still more in the suggestion that God Himself demanded it. We all despise the man who demands continued assurance of his own virtue, intelligence or delightfulness; we despise still more the crowd of people round every dictator, every millionaire, every celebrity, who gratify that demand. Thus a picture, at once ludicrous and horrible, both of God and of His worshippers, threatened to appear in my mind … I did not see that it is in the process

41

of being worshipped that God communicates His presence to men.

It is in the process of worshipping that we will learn from God and will be transformed, for "we all, who with unveiled faces contemplate the Lord's glory, are being transformed into his image with ever-increasing glory, which comes from the Lord, who is the Spirit" (2 Cor. 3:18). If we want to be more like Jesus, we need to take time to behold the beauty of the Lord and worship Him.

Oswald Chambers was a prominent Christian minister and teacher. He was best known as the author of the widely read devotional *My Utmost for His Highest*. He was born in Scotland in 1874 and died in Egypt 1917 as the result of a ruptured appendix because he suffered the extreme pain of appendicitis for three days, refusing to take a hospital bed needed by wounded soldiers. He used to teach, "Worshipping God is the great essential for fitness. If you have not been worshipping … when you get into work you will not only be useless yourself, but a tremendous hindrance to those that are associated with you." Dear friends, to be able to be good husbands, good wives, good parents, or good professionals, we need to spend time dwelling in the presence of the Lord.

Another influential writer and preacher of the last century was the American A. W. Tozer (1897–1963). He said,

> Man was made to worship God. God gave to man a harp and said, here above all the creatures that I have made and created I have given you the largest harp. I put more strings on your instrument and I

have given you a wider range than I have given to any other creature. You can worship me in a manner that no other creature can, And when he sinned man took that instrument and threw it down in the mud and there it has lain for centuries, rusted, broken, unstrung; and man, instead of playing a harp like the angels and seeking to worship God in all of his activities, is ego-centered and turns in on himself and sulks and swears and laughs and sings, but it's all without joy and without worship ... Worship is the missing jewel in modern evangelicalism. We're organized; we work; we have our agendas. We have almost everything, but there's one thing that the churches, even the gospel churches, do not have: that is the ability to worship. We are not cultivating the art of worship. It's the one shinning gem that is lost to the modern church, and I believe that we ought to search for this until we find it.

So what is worship? Mr. Joseph S. Carroll, founder of the Evangelical Institute of Greenville, South Carolina, wrote a book on *How to Worship Jesus Christ* where he teaches that the word *worship* comes from *Weorth-scipe* (an Anglo-Saxon word) that means the worth ship—to ascribe the worth or to attribute worth to the One you worship [12].

He also teaches that the attitude of worship is an attitude of submission. In the last book of the Bible, Revelation, when the

---

[12]   J.S Carroll, How to Worship Jesus Christ, Great Comission, Greenville, SC, 1984

apostle John had a vision of heaven, he describes what he saw this way:

> The twenty-four elders fall down before him who sits on the throne and worship him who lives for ever and ever. They lay their crowns before the throne and say: You are worthy, our Lord and God, to receive glory and honor and power, for you created all things, and by your will they were created and have their being. (Rev. 4:10–11)

To fall down before a person is an attitude of complete submission. The Hebrews would fall flat, face on the floor before the one they worshipped. Submission is the first essential quality of worship. The purpose of the crown is to draw attention to the one wearing it, to exalt the wearer. But worshippers of Jesus Christ cast their crowns before the feet of the one on the throne, saying, "Only you, oh Lord, are worthy to receive all honor and glory."

When Count von Zinzendorf (1700–1760) was a young man, he visited an art gallery in Düsseldorf, Germany. As he admired the various priceless paintings, he was suddenly transfixed by one called *Ecce Homo* (Behold the Man) by Domínico Feti. As the curator of the art gallery made his rounds, he noticed this young man gazing intently at that painting hour after hour. Finally, when it came time to close the gallery, the young count was still there. At last the curator went to him, putting his hand on his shoulder, and was about to tell him that he must leave when he saw tears streaming down the young man's cheeks. There in front of Count von Zinzendorf was a magnificent painting of the slain Lamb of God, beneath which were the words, "All this I did for thee, what has thou done for me?" Before that painting of the crucified Christ, the Holy Spirit spoke, and Nicolaus von Zinzendorf from that day had a broken heart[13]—broken from self and offered up to God. Although he became the king's judicial counselor at Dresden, he lost all interest in worldly things and decided to serve God. He received in his lands the refugees from Moravia and formed the Herrhut (The Lord's Watch) a Christian community of which it is said that sent more missionaries in twenty years than the whole of protestant church in the first two hundred years.

The second reason why David wanted to dwell in the house of the Lord was to seek Him in His temple. He desired to seek, to ask, to pursue, to enquire, to go after, to listen, and to meditate in the Lord. He wanted to be with Him. He wanted to learn from Him. He wanted to know Him. It is not passing by and getting a glimpse or a quick look in a hurry. To dwell, to behold, to enquire, and to meditate all take time; actually, it takes forever. Have you seen a couple in love? Their thoughts are on the beloved all the time: *What is she doing now? What is he thinking? What does she like? How can I please him?* When together, they want to be together, forever. We know they are in love. David was in love with the Lord. He was his only desire and only purpose in life.

Brother Lawrence was a French monk (Carmelite) (1611–1691). Although a humble cook, he continually lived in the presence of God while working in his monastery's kitchen. The

---

[13]   J.S Carroll, How to Worship Jesus Christ, Great Comission, Greenville, SC, 1984

most trivial thing he did was done unto the Lord. He was able to turn even the most common tasks—like preparing meals and washing dishes—into acts of praise and communion with God. The key to friendship with God, he said, is not changing what you do but changing your attitude toward what you do. What you normally do for yourself, you begin doing for God, whether it is eating, bathing, working, relaxing, or taking out the trash.

It is said that people could feel the presence of God in his kitchen because it was a sanctuary where he met and worshipped his Lord. Rick Warren, in his devotionals, said that today we often feel we must "get away" from our daily routine to worship God, but that is only because we haven't learned to practice His presence all the time. Brother Lawrence found it easy to worship God through the common tasks of life; he didn't have to go away for special spiritual retreats. This is what Adam and Eve had in the garden of Eden. Worship was not an event to attend but a perpetual attitude. They were in constant communion with God. Certainly it is very important to have special times set aside to seek the Lord and worship Him together, as we do every Sunday, but we can continue in His presence daily in our homes, in our offices, wherever we go.

When we worship, we will be doing what the Westminster declaration said: "Man's chief end is to glorify God and to enjoy him forever." And this is also what we will be doing throughout all eternity in heaven—to admire, to behold, to dwell with, and to enjoy our Savior and Lord forever.

I would like to close this section with a story of two sisters.

As Jesus and his disciples were on their way, he came to a village where a woman named Martha opened her home to him. She had a sister called Mary, who sat at the Lord's feet listening to what he said. But Martha was distracted by all the preparations that had to be made. She came to him and asked, "Lord, don't you care that my sister has left me to do the work by myself? Tell her to help me!" "Martha, Martha," the Lord answered, "you are worried and upset about many things, but few things are needed—or indeed only one. Mary has chosen what is better, and it will not be taken away from her." (Luke 10:38–42)

Many times we are like Martha, worried and upset about many things. Why not learn with Mary to stop running to please the world. We must stop trying to fill the holes in our heart that only God can fill. We don't need to prove anything to anybody. Listen to Jesus saying, "Few things are needed—or indeed only one." Are we missing the only one thing that really is needed?

St. Augustine in his *Confessions* said, "God, you have made us for yourself, and our hearts are restless till they find their rest in you." [14]

There is a beautiful hymn by Horatius Bonar (1808–1889), Scottish pastor and writer, called "I Heard the Voice of Jesus Say." It says,

---

[14] Saint Augustine. (354–430). The Confessions of St. Augustine. The First Book. The Harvard Classics. 1909–14.

I heard the voice of Jesus say, "Come unto Me and rest;
Lay down, thou weary one, lay down Thy head upon
    My breast."
I came to Jesus as I was, weary and worn and sad;
I found in Him a resting place, and He has made
    me glad.

I heard the voice of Jesus say, "Behold, I freely give
The living water; thirsty one, stoop down, and drink,
    and live."
I came to Jesus, and I drank of that life giving stream;
My thirst was quenched, my soul revived, and now I
    live in Him.

I heard the voice of Jesus say, "I am this dark world's
    light;
Look unto Me, thy morn shall rise, and all thy day
    be bright."
I looked to Jesus, and I found in Him my star, my sun;
And in that light of life I'll walk, till traveling days
    are done.

Prayer

Dear Jesus, thank You for Your calling. "Come to me, all who labor and are heavy laden, and I will give you rest" (Matt. 11:27–30). We come today with many worries and burdens, things we cannot handle ourselves. We need You. Help us, Lord to sit still at Your feet, to listen, to dwell in Your presence, to behold Your beauty, and to focus on the only one thing that is needed—to seek what David and Mary were looking for. Help us, *Lord,* to rest in You

The Passover Lamb

When I came to China in 2008, it was just after Chinese New Year. I was amazed to see so many red decorations and designs in the front doors of the houses. I learned that an ancient legend says that this celebration started when a mythological beast called *nian* attacked the villages, destroying the crops and eating their children. But one day they saw the beast was scared away by a little child wearing red. They discovered that nian was afraid of this color, so they decided to cover their front doors with red lanterns and lots of red decorations. It is said that from that day on, nian never came to the village again. This became the most popular and celebrated festival in the Chinese culture. I could not avoid seeing a parallel in the Jewish culture's Passover, which is celebrated also in the early spring, when the people of Israel covered their doorposts with red to protect them from the destroyer that killed all the firstborn sons in the country. The difference is that in the Passover, what was painted in the door was the blood of a little lamb. Let's go through the Bible and meditate on the Passover Lamb. The first Passover happened when the Israelites were slaves in Egypt, and God heard their cry, sending Moses to deliver them.

> The Lord said to Moses and Aaron in Egypt, "This month is to be for you the first month, the first month

of your year. Tell the whole community of Israel that on the tenth day of this month each man is to take a lamb for his family, one for each household. ... The animals you choose must be year-old males without defect, and you may take them from the sheep or the goats. Take care of them until the fourteenth day of the month, when all the members of the community of Israel must slaughter them at twilight. Then they are to take some of the blood and put it on the sides and tops of the doorframes of the houses where they eat the lambs. That same night they are to eat the meat roasted over the fire, along with bitter herbs, and bread made without yeast. ... This is how you are to eat it: with your cloak tucked into your belt, your sandals on your feet and your staff in your hand. Eat it in haste; it is the Lord's Passover. ... Then Moses summoned all the elders of Israel and said to them, "Go at once and select the animals for your families and slaughter the Passover lamb. Take a bunch of hyssop, dip it into the blood in the basin and put some of the blood on the top and on both sides of the doorframe. None of you shall go out of the door of your house until morning. When the Lord goes through the land to strike down the Egyptians, he will see the blood on the top and sides of the doorframe and will pass over that doorway, and he will not permit the destroyer to enter your houses and strike you down." (Ex. 12:1–23)

The Lord saw the blood on the top and sides of the doorframe and passed over that doorway (hence the name of the holiday) and did not permit the destroyer to enter their houses. Passover was a celebration of deliverance from death in that terrible night and also a celebration of deliverance from slavery. They were made free in that same night. It was a step of faith and dependence on God and on the blood of an innocent, perfect, precious little Lamb.

If we go back in time to the first book of the Bible, we will find that the patriarch Abraham also met a lamb. In Genesis 22 it is written:

> Sometime later God tested Abraham. He said to him, "Abraham!" "Here I am," he replied. Then God said, "Take your son, your only son, whom you love— Isaac—and go to the region of Moriah. Sacrifice him there as a burnt offering on a mountain I will show you." Early the next morning Abraham got up and loaded his donkey. He took with him two of his servants and his son Isaac. When he had cut enough wood for the burnt offering, he set out for the place God had told him about. On the third day Abraham looked up and saw the place in the distance. He said to his servants, "Stay here with the donkey while I and the boy go over there. We will worship and then we will come back to you." Abraham took the wood for the burnt offering and placed it on his son Isaac, and he himself carried the fire and the knife. As the two of them went on together, Isaac spoke up and said to his father Abraham, "Father?" "Yes, my son?" Abraham replied. "The fire and wood are here," Isaac said, "but where is the lamb for the burnt offering?" Abraham answered, "God himself will provide the

lamb for the burnt offering, my son." And the two of them went on together. When they reached the place God had told him about, Abraham built an altar there and arranged the wood on it. He bound his son Isaac and laid him on the altar, on top of the wood. Then he reached out his hand and took the knife to slay his son. But the angel of the Lord called out to him from heaven, "Abraham! Abraham!" "Here I am," he replied. "Do not lay a hand on the boy," he said. "Do not do anything to him. Now I know that you fear God, because you have not withheld from me your son, your only son." Abraham looked up and there in a thicket he saw a ram caught by its horns. He went over and took the ram and sacrificed it as a burnt offering instead of his son. So Abraham called that place The Lord Will Provide. And to this day it is said, "On the mountain of the Lord it will be provided."

This episode in Abraham's life shows the unimaginable cost of his sacrifice. Much more than his own life, it was his son, the son of a promise that he had waited for until he was one hundred years old. Isaac his only son, whom he loved.

A tradition that first appears in Josephus, and that is now almost universally accepted, asserts that "the land of Moriah" of Genesis, the very spot of the sacrifice of Isaac, is the same "Mount Moriah" of the Chronicles, the spot on which Jehovah appeared to David and on which the temple was built in Jerusalem.[15]

---

[15]   W. Smith, *Smith's Bible Names Dictionary*, Grand Rapids, MI: Christian Classics Ethereal Library Publisher, Year1884.

The temple was central in the life of Israel. In its most inner part was a cubic room separated by a thick curtain called the most holy place. It was a meeting place for God and man, but only the high priest could enter there just once a year on the Atonement Day. In this room there was an ark covered with gold called the ark of covenant. The cover of the ark was called the mercy seat or atonement cover, in Hebrew *hilasterion* or propitiatory, meaning the sacrifice that atones or appeases the wrath of God [16]. It was a clear lesson that sin is not a light matter for God, "for the wages of sin is death" (Rom. 6:23). The high priest on the Atonement Day would enter the Most Holy Place through the curtain with the blood of a lamb. He would sprinkle it on top of the cover of the ark and confess his sins first and then the sins of his people. The blood would show that the penalty of their sins was paid for with the death of an innocent, substitutionary, precious lamb.

Between the Old and the New Testament there is a period of silence. There was no prophetic voice, no message from God. People wondered, "Why does God not speak to us anymore?" But after four hundred years, a prophet called John the Baptist appeared preaching in the Jordan River, "Repent, for the kingdom of God is near. Then went out to him Jerusalem, and all Judea, and all the region round about Jordan" (Matt. 3:1–6).

The next day John saw Jesus coming toward him and said, "Look, the Lamb of God, who takes away the sin of the world!" (John 1:29). This is the one the whole of Israel's history pointed to, the real Lamb of God who takes away the sin of the world.

---

16 W.E.Vine, An Expository Dictionary of Biblical Words, Thomas Nelson Publisher, Nashville TN, 1984

After three years of ministry, teaching, serving, and loving, one day

> when Jesus had finished saying all these things, he said to his disciples, "As you know, the Passover is two days away—and the Son of Man will be handed over to be crucified." (Matt. 26:1–2)

Two days later, exactly on the Passover day, Jesus was stripped naked, bitten, mocked, and spit upon. They put a crown of thorns on His head and sent Him to the cross, which for the Romans was the most cruel and hideous form of torture and death, reserved only for the worst criminals, and which for the Jews meant above all a curse from God (Deut. 21:23). Three of the strongest soldiers would strike thirteen times each with a leather whip woven with pieces of bone and metal.

Eusebius describes that in this process the veins, muscles, and even bones and bowels were exposed. Then the wrists were nailed to the cross. His knees were bent out for both ankles to be nailed between the tibia and the Achilles tendon with a single long nail. For Jesus it was not only the physical pain and emotional distress of rejection and shame, but above all He suffered the weight of our sins and the spiritual separation from God that caused the most suffering. At the cross He didn't call for His Father as He always did, but "My God, my God, why have you forsaken me?" This is because, at that moment He was taking our place, He was carrying our sins. He received upon Himself like a lightning rod all the immeasurable power of the lightning of the wrath of the holy God against our sin.

In 700 BC, Isaiah prophesied about Him.

> He took up our infirmities and carried our sorrows, yet we considered him punished by God, stricken by him, and afflicted. But he was pierced for our transgressions, he was crushed for our iniquities; the punishment that brought us peace was upon him, and by his wounds we are healed ... The Lord has laid on him the iniquity of us all. He was oppressed and afflicted, yet he did not open his mouth; he was led like a lamb to the slaughter, and as a sheep before her shearers is silent, so he did not open his mouth. (Isa. 53)

Matthew Henry comments that it is

> Jesus Christ the Son of the Father, one anointed by the Father for the whole office of mediation, for that of the intercessor or advocate. It is Jesus Christ the righteous, the righteous one in the court and sight of the Judge. But here the clients are guilty; their innocence and legal righteousness cannot be pleaded; their sin must be confessed or supposed. It is the advocate's own righteousness that he must plead for the criminals. He has been righteous to the death, righteous for them; he has brought in everlasting righteousness. This the Judge will not deny. Upon this score he pleads, that the clients' sins may not be imputed to them. And he is the propitiation for our sins, 1 John 2:2. He is the expiatory victim, the propitiatory sacrifice that has

been offered to the Judge for all our offences against his majesty, and law, and government[17].

Jesus is the lawyer who paid Himself the penalty we deserved and died that we may live. "We have an advocate with the Father—Jesus Christ, the Righteous One. He is the atoning sacrifice for our sins, and not only for ours but also for the sins of the whole world" (1 John 2:1–2).

Two thousand years after Abraham, in a little hill rounded like a bare skull called Golgotha or Calvary (*Easton's Bible Dictionary*), nearby Mount Moriah, God "did not spare his own Son, but gave him up" as a sacrifice in the cross for us all. The cross is where the immensity of the justice of God met the immensity of His love.

At 3:00 in the afternoon, Jesus said, "It is finished." "With that, he bowed his head and gave up his spirit" (John 19:30). Finished in Greek is *tetelestai*, and it means accomplished, executed, completed, concluded, expired, covered, or debt discharged.[18] All the debts of our sins were paid for, covered completely, nothing left, tetelestai, finished, it is done, mission accomplished, executed, and completed forever.

> At that moment the curtain of the temple was torn in two from top to bottom. The earth shook, the rocks split and the tombs broke open. … When the centurion and those with him who were guarding Jesus saw the earthquake and all that had happened,

---

17   Matthew Henry Commentary, on http://www.biblegateway.com

18   *Strong's Exhaustive Concordance of the Bible*, 5055.

they were terrified, and exclaimed, "Surely he was the Son of God!" (Matt. 27:50–54)

In the moment Jesus died, the thick curtain that separated the Most Holy Place in the temple was torn from top to bottom. That barrier—the wall sin built between us and God—was removed completely as always an initiative of God toward men. Jesus opened up the way.

> Therefore, brothers and sisters, since we have confidence to enter the Most Holy Place by the blood of Jesus, by a new and living way opened for us through the curtain, that is, his body, and since we have a great priest over the house of God, let us draw near to God with a sincere heart and with the full assurance that faith brings, having our hearts sprinkled to cleanse us from a guilty conscience and having our bodies washed with pure water. (Heb. 10:19–22)

> "Come now, let us settle the matter," says the Lord. "Though your sins are like scarlet, they shall be as white as snow; though they are red as crimson, they shall be like wool." (Isa. 1:18)

The almighty God is inviting you, "Come, now, let us settle the matter. All your sins will be forgiven, forgotten, forever." This is grace, undeserved favor, and a priceless gift. Isaac Watts wrote three hundred years ago:

When I survey the wondrous cross
On which the Prince of glory died,
My richest gain I count but loss,
And pour contempt on all my pride.

Forbid it, Lord, that I should boast,
Save in the death of Christ my God!
All the vain things that charm me most,
I sacrifice them to His blood.

See from His head, His hands, His feet,
Sorrow and love flow mingled down!
Did e'er such love and sorrow meet,
Or thorns compose so rich a crown?

Were the whole realm of nature mine,
That were a present far too small;
Love so amazing, so divine,
Demands my soul, my life, my all.[19]

But the good news does not end here. On the third day:

> After the Sabbath, at dawn on the first day of the
> week, Mary Magdalene and the other Mary went to
> look at the tomb. There was a violent earthquake, for
> an angel of the Lord came down from heaven and,
> going to the tomb, rolled back the stone and sat on
> it. His appearance was like lightning, and his clothes
> were white as snow. The guards were so afraid of him

---

[19] When I Survey the Wondrous Cross," an Easter hymn by Isaac Watts,1707.
See Songsandhymns.org for more about this and other Easter hymns.

that they shook and became like dead men. The angel said to the women, "Do not be afraid, for I know that you are looking for Jesus, who was crucified. He is not here; he has risen, just as he said. Come and see the place where he lay. Then go quickly and tell his disciples: 'He has risen from the dead and is going ahead of you into Galilee. There you will see him.' Now I have told you." So the women hurried away from the tomb, afraid yet filled with joy, and ran to tell his disciples. Suddenly Jesus met them. "Greetings," he said. They came to him, clasped his feet and worshiped him. Then Jesus said to them, "Do not be afraid. Go and tell my brothers to go to Galilee; there they will see me." (Matt. 28:1–10)

Then the eleven disciples went to Galilee, to the mountain where Jesus had told them to go. When they saw him, they worshiped him; but some doubted. Then Jesus came to them and said, "All authority in heaven and on earth has been given to me. Therefore go and make disciples of all nations, baptizing them in the name of the Father and of the Son and of the Holy Spirit, and teaching them to obey everything I have commanded you. And surely I am with you always, to the very end of the age." (Matt. 28:16–20)

The Lord Jesus, rose from the dead as a sign that His sacrifice was accepted and bestowed with all authority in heaven and on earth. He gave the disciples a commission—the great commission—to go and make disciples of all nations. And so they did. These simple fishermen of Galilee, without formal education and without money but filled with the Holy Spirit, faithfully spread the good news of salvation, of forgiveness, of hope, and of the love of God wherever they went. In thirty years, it spread throughout the whole Roman empire. They even reached Caesar's house. They were persecuted, put in prison, and killed, but nothing could stop the living Word of God. It crossed oceans and went on to Europe, to America, to Africa, to Asia, and to the uttermost parts of the world. That is why we are here today—because someone, a friend or a family member—told us about Jesus. And the same commission is given to us today to go and tell what God has done for you. Jesus gave us a promise: "I am with you always, to the very end of the age."

Passover is the week when we remember the death and resurrection of Jesus Christ and His victory over sin. This is good news that is free for all people because of Jesus. I wish that not only everyone in China but the whole world would find a shelter under the blood of the Lamb. One day, when we enter the very presence of the living God all His people will rejoice. When the apostle John had a vision of heaven, he wrote,

> After this I looked, and there before me was a great multitude that no one could count, from every nation, tribe, people and language, standing before the throne and before the Lamb. They were wearing white robes and were holding palm branches in their hands. And they cried out in a loud voice: "Salvation belongs to our God, who sits on the throne, and to the Lamb." All the angels were standing around the throne

and around the elders and the four living creatures. They fell down on their faces before the throne and worshiped God, saying: "Amen! Praise and glory and wisdom and thanks and honor and power and strength be to our God for ever and ever. Amen!" Then one of the elders asked me, "These in white robes—who are they, and where did they come from?" I answered, "Sir, you know." And he said, "These are they who have come out of the great tribulation; they have washed their robes and made them white in the blood of the Lamb. Therefore, they are before the throne of God and serve him day and night in his temple; and he who sits on the throne will shelter them with his presence. Never again will they hunger; never again will they thirst. 'The sun will not beat down on them,' nor any scorching heat. For the Lamb at the center of the throne will be their shepherd; he will lead them to springs of living water. And God will wipe away every tear from their eyes. (Rev. 7:9–17)

Prayer

Dear Father, we thank You for the privilege to be part of Your wonderful redemptive plan. Thank You, Father, for loving us so much that You gave Your only Son, who died that we may live. Help us, Lord, that we may live this life in a way that is worthy of Your love.

Remain in Me

When I first came to Shanghai as a family doctor, I saw a little American girl (who was maybe four or five years old) who came to the clinic with stomach pain. As I was pressing her abdomen, I asked, "Is it painful?"

Then I looked at the mother's face, and I saw an expression of incredulity and concern as she said, "She does not know that word." She asked the child. "Is it hurting, honey?"

After the visit I thought to myself, *Why did I come to China? I am not Chinese, and I don't speak Chinese. I am a Japanese descendant, but I don't speak Japanese as a native Japanese. I don't speak English as a native English speaker. I don't even know children's language. What am I doing here?*

There are times in life when we face crises. They can be relationships at work, in the family, or an identity crisis. We may be asking ourselves, "Who am I after all? What should I do?" The disciples were facing such a time. They had left their jobs to follow Jesus. They placed their hope in the Messiah, but now their leader and master would be leaving shortly. Actually, He would die on a cross, and they would face persecution from their own people. It was a time of uncertainty, worry, and confusion. Jesus took time to encourage and prepare them. He had a private meeting with His disciples prior to His crucifixion, and John described it in five chapters, from 13:1 to 17:26.

This section begins with an account of Jesus washing the disciples' feet. Almighty God took the position of a humble servant, gave them an example, and said, "Now that I, your Lord and Teacher, have washed your feet, you also should wash one another's feet." Then there is a lengthy section known as the farewell discourse, which consists of teachings for the disciples (13:31–16:33) and a concluding prayer by Jesus for them (17:1–26).

One of the teachings in this section is called the vine and the branches. It says,

> I am the true vine, and my Father is the gardener. He cuts off every branch in me that bears no fruit, while every branch that does bear fruit he prunes so that it will be even more fruitful. You are already clean because of the word I have spoken to you. Remain in me, as I also remain in you. No branch can bear fruit by itself; it must remain in the vine. Neither can you bear fruit unless you remain in me. I am the vine; you are the branches. If you remain in me and I in you, you will bear much fruit; apart from me you can do nothing. If you do not remain in me, you are like a branch that is thrown away and withers; such branches are picked up, thrown into the fire and burned. If you remain in me and my words remain in you, ask whatever you wish, and it will be done for you. This is to my Father's glory, that you bear much fruit, showing yourselves to be my disciples. As the Father has loved me, so have I loved you. Now remain in my love. If you keep my commands, you

> will remain in my love, just as I have kept my Father's commands and remain in his love. I have told you this so that my joy may be in you and that your joy may be complete. My command is this: Love each other as I have loved you. Greater love has no one than this: to lay down one's life for one's friends. You are my friends if you do what I command. I no longer call you servants, because a servant does not know his master's business. Instead, I have called you friends, for everything that I learned from my Father I have made known to you. You did not choose me, but I chose you and appointed you so that you might go and bear fruit—fruit that will last—and so that whatever you ask in my name the Father will give you. This is my command: Love each other. (John 15:1–17)

Intervarsity Press observes that this is not a parable since is not a story but rather an extended metaphor (Carson 1991:513) [20] or basically an allegory, for all the details have significance. The main point of the image is clear enough: the intimate union of believers with Jesus.

Jesus is teaching us three lessons in this text.

1. "I am the true vine"
The vines of Palestine were celebrated both for luxuriant growth and for the immense clusters of grapes they produced, which were sometimes carried on a staff between two men, as in the case

---

[20]   http://www.biblegateway.com

of the spies into the Promised Land (Num. 13:23).[21] They were used to produce wine, which was considered a symbol of joy and happiness.

One of the characteristics of the vine is that it is not a lofty, upright tree that can be reached only if we are strong and agile to be able to climb high to find its fruits. The vine is a tree that bends itself, that comes down so it is near to the ground and available to anyone who desires. Actually, we need to humble ourselves to be able to find its fruit.

When Moses asked God his name in Exodus 3, He said "I am who I am" and "This is what you are to say to the Israelites: 'I am has sent me to you.'"

Matthew Henry (1662–1714) comments:

> His name denotes what he is in himself, and signifies,
> (1.) That he is self-existent; he has his being of himself,
> and has no dependence upon any other. Being self-
> existent, he cannot but be self-sufficient, and therefore
> all-sufficient, and the inexhaustible fountain of being
> and bliss. (2.) That he is eternal and unchangeable,
> and always the same, yesterday, to-day, and for ever;
> he will be what he will be and what he is; (3.) That
> this is such a name as checks all bold and curious
> enquiries concerning God. Let it suffice us to know
> that he is what he is, what he ever was, and ever will
> be. (4.) That he is faithful and true to all his promises,

---

21   W. Smith, *Smith's Bible Names Dictionary*, Grand Rapids, MI: Christian Classics Ethereal Library Publisher, Year1884.

unchangeable in his word as well as in his nature. Let
Israel know this, I AM hath sent me unto you.

This is the God who eternally is, that always was, and always will be. He is the fountain of all existence, immutable, unchangeable, whose name is so holy that the scribes didn't dare to pronounce it because they were not worthy to utter it with unclean lips. Nobody knew how to read the holy name, for in the Hebrew Bible it was written with four consonants only, YHWH, called the tetragrammaton. It was transliterated as Yahweh or Jehovah, intercalating the vowels of Adonai or Lord, but nobody knows exactly how to read the name of God. How can we read a name or a word without vowels?

But this is the "I am" who reveals Himself to us in the book of John as, "I am the door, I am the way, I am the truth and the life, I am the good shepherd, I am the living water, I am the light of the world, and here as I am the true vine." This reveals God in a way that we can understand and relate to. We can know Him and find in Him the Way, the Truth, the abundant Life, the water to quench the thirst of our souls, and the Good Shepherd who loved us so much that gave His life to save us.

Although He is the transcendent, unattainable, unsearchable, indescribable God, He is also God with us who made Himself nothing, taking the very nature of a servant, being made in human likeness. And being found in appearance as a man, humbled himself and became obedient to death—even death on a cross! Jesus is the heavenly vine that was planted on Earth, the only source of real joy, abundant life, and overflowing love. He is the only one who can say with full meaning of each word, "I am the true vine." Do you know Him?

2. *"My Father is the gardener."*
The image of a gardener is not of someone sitting in his office who is well-dressed and looking the garden from the window. It is somebody who is working all day outside who is sweaty and has muddy hands, taking care of each plant in the garden personally.

My grandfather was a farmer. He bought a piece of land in an island called *Ilha Bela* (or Beautiful Island) in Brazil about seventy years ago. He planted all kinds of trees—mango, orange, vine, litchi, guava—and all kinds of ornamental trees, flowers, and vegetables. He used to wake up with the first cockcrow, listen the news on the radio, and eat his breakfast. When the sun started to rise, he would go up the mountain to take care of the property.

As children, my sisters and I used to spend our summer and winter breaks with Grandpa and grandma. Many times we went with him up the mountain, playing around while Grandpa was working. From time to time, he would stop to drink some water, wipe the sweat from his face, and sit by a rock, watching the ocean beneath and the sky above. Sometimes he needed to remove the weeds all around the property to protect from fire that came from outside. Sometimes he would wake up at night and with a torch would look for the track of sauva, which is a kind of ant that could destroy the whole plantation in a night. But his delight was to bring the fruit of his work to the table: beautiful tomatoes, carrots, corn, mangoes, and bananas. He worked hard, but above all he loved that place. He enjoyed his garden until the last minute of his ninety-four years of life.

In the same way, our Father is not only the Designer of the universe, to whom all belongs, but He is also actively involved in the affairs of this world, caring for each one of us individually. It is enough to know that the Father is the gardener. He is in charge, He is in control, and we can rest assured like a baby in her mother's arms.

Jesus is teaching also that there are two things that the gardener does concerning the branches: to cut off and to prune. He cuts off every branch that bears no fruit because if the branch is just externally, mechanically there but does not have a real life connection with the vine, it should not be there. If there is a vital and spiritual connection, it should bear fruit. The question we need to ask ourselves and make sure is, are we really connected to Jesus? Physical presence, intellectual assent, and external appearances are not enough. Real spiritual intimacy with Jesus is a must. This is the most important question in life because the answer will define our eternal destiny.

Every branch that does bear fruit, He prunes, so the vine will be even more fruitful. We need to say that this branch bears fruit not because of its own merit but simply because it is connected to the vine, for there is no other way to bear fruit unless it is united to the source of life. Pruning means cleaning, removing parts that are not appropriate, unnecessary, and excessive, with the purpose of making the branch more healthy, more light, and more fruitful. It may be painful, but is necessary. It is said that suffering is the university of God. We learn many things from suffering. Paul spent three years in the desert, and Moses spent forty years alone with God. But it was there that they learned to depend on Him, to trust Him, and to develop intimacy with God. We may not know why many things happen to us, but if we come to a closer, deeper, and stronger relationship with the Lord, it will bring invaluable blessings to our lives.

3. "You are the branch."
The vine is the very source of strength, energy, and life for the branch. The branch cannot do anything apart from the vine. The moment it separates from the vine, the branch will wither and die. In the same way, apart from Jesus, the more we try, the more we will get tired, frustrated, and discouraged because we don't have in ourselves the energy to live the lives we were designed to live.

It is like a machine that was designed to use a magnificent and pure source of energy but lost connection with this source of power and is using a temporary battery that allows it to move for a while but not as it should. But if it is connected again to the original source of power, it will work perfectly to its full potential. Can we be kind, faithful, and gentle all the time? Can we never get angry, lose our temper, or fail to love as we should? That is why Jesus said, "Remain in Me. Without Me you can do nothing."

This is easy to forget. We experience so much busyness in this life, pressures in work, and so many worldly affairs and forces to pull us apart. We have the tendency to think we are the boss or the person in charge. We think we need to fix the world all by ourselves, apart from God. Jesus says, "No! Your only responsibility is to remain connected to the vine. Everything else is taken care off." Jesus repeats no less than eleven times in this passage the word *remain* because remaining is a must and is the secret to fruitfulness.

> Remain in me, as I also remain in you. No branch can bear fruit by itself; it must remain in the vine. Neither can you bear fruit unless you remain in me. I am the vine; you are the branches. If you remain in me and I in you, you will bear much fruit; apart from me you can do nothing. If you do not remain in me, you are like a branch that is thrown away and withers; ... If you remain in me and my words remain in you, ask whatever you wish, and it will be done for you. As the Father has loved me, so have I loved you. Now remain in my love. If you keep my commands, you will remain in my love, just as I have kept my Father's commands and remain in his love. My command is this: Love each other as I have loved you. Greater love has no one than this: to lay down one's life for one's friends. (John 15:)

We learn from the Bible that God the Father, the Son, and the Holy Spirit live in a wonderful relationship of love for all eternity. One day God took the initiative to create the world and human beings to include us in His love. He sent His Son to become flesh, taking our human nature so we may become like Him, partaking in His divine nature. Jesus said, "As the Father has loved me, so have I loved you. Now remain in my love" and "Love each other as I have loved you." It is like a happy family dancing and hugging each other and including and embracing more and more people until it becomes a really big family from every nation of the world.

Prof. Luiz Sayao from Brazil spoke on the family, telling us that we live in a world that is characterized by its struggle for power in the family, in business, in traffic, in politics—everywhere. We are taught that we need to be the head, not the tail, even pushing others aside. But Jesus showed us a different way of life, a different power: the power of love. Love is so powerful that cannot be defeated. It wins and conquers not by egocentric authority but by respect and submission. But the proof of true love is the willingness to die for the other person.

When my daughter Grace was four years old, she suddenly asked me, "Daddy, would you die for me?" To this day, I don't know from where she got this question, but this is the question that shows the real love. "For God demonstrates his own love for us in this: While we were still sinners, Christ died for us" (Rom. 5:8).

"Remain in me, as I also remain in you. If you remain in me and my words remain in you, ask whatever you wish, and it will be done for you. Remain in my love. I have told you this so that my joy may be in you and that your joy may be complete." We are in Jesus, and Jesus in us. His Word is in us, we are in His love, and His joy is in us. This is relationship, connection, dependency, and intimacy.

Have you ever seeing a vine? Many times it is difficult to distinguish the trunk from the branches. They are intertwined, mingled; they are one. This is what Jesus wants—an intimate relationship with us. His love, His joy, His Word—He in us and we in Him. The consequence of this union is that whatever we ask in His name, the Father will give because our will will be His will. The Father will be glorified, and we will show we are His disciples.

To be a Christian is not just learning some doctrine or signing up to be a member of a group. To be a Christian is a vital, personal relationship with the living God through Jesus Christ. It is a connection of life. We are like a branch that was dying, withering, but was graciously connected to the vine. Now we receive a new sap of life, of love, of joy that comes from Him. There is a new energy within and strength to grow and produce fruit. Are you in a living relationship with Jesus and connected with Him? If you are already connected with Jesus, you just need to remain there and rest in Him. The fruit that comes out when we are connected to Jesus is no other but love, joy, peace, forbearance, kindness, goodness, faithfulness, gentleness, and self-control (Gal. 5:22–23), which are the fruits of the Spirit—fruits of His divine nature.

"You did not choose me, but I chose you and appointed you so that you might go and bear fruit—fruit that will last." What a privilege to be chosen by Jesus to go and bear fruit and fruit that will last. And the best of all is that our part in this is just remaining in Him. We must lean and depend on, nothing more than resting in Jesus. In the book *Abide in Christ*, Andrew Murray (1828–1917), a South African writer, teacher, and pastor, comments[22].

Beautiful image of the believer abiding in Christ! He
not only grows in strength, the union with the Vine

---

[22]   A. Murray, Abide in Christ, Whitaker House, 2002, first published in 1972

becoming ever surer and firmer, he also bears fruit,
yea, much fruit. ... He is in his circle a centre of life
and of blessing, and that simply because he abides in
Christ, and receives from Him the Spirit and the life
of which he can impart to others. ... As surely as the
branch abiding in a fruitful vine bears fruit, so surely,
yea, much more surely, will a soul abiding in Christ
be made a blessing.

The reason of this is easily understood. If Christ, the
heavenly Vine, has taken the believer as a branch,
then He has pledged Himself, in the very nature of
things, to supply the sap and spirit and nourishment
to make it bring forth fruit. ... The soul need but have
one care,—to abide closely, fully, wholly. He will give
the fruit.

Abiding in Jesus you come into contact with His
infinite love; its fire begins to burn within your heart;
you see the beauty of love; ... As you are more closely
united to Him, somewhat of that passion for souls
which urged Him to Calvary begins to breathe within
you, and you are ready to follow His footsteps, to
forsake the heaven of your own happiness, and devote
your life to win the souls Christ has taught you to
love. The very spirit of the Vine is love; the spirit of
love streams into the branch that abides in Him.

One of the first biographies I read after becoming a Christian
was of Hudson Taylor, who was born in England in1832 and
died in Chansha, Hunan province, in 1905. During the early

years in China, facing many financial and health difficulties and persecution, he was struggling when the Lord gave him the words of John 15: "I am the vine; you are the branches. If you remain in me and I in you, you will bear much fruit; apart from me you can do nothing." He learned to rest in the assurance that his sole responsibility was to remain in Christ.

After fifty-one years of ministry in China, he led one hundred and twenty-five thousand people to faith and is considered the father of modern missions. What was the secret of his lifelong and effective ministry? His son and daughter-in-law who travelled with him in his later years said that frequently after riding a spring-less cart for many hours, they would find an inn, which was just a large room where everybody slept together. Even as an aged man, just before dawn there would be a scratching of a match, the lighting of a candle, and Hudson Taylor would worship God. It was said that even before the sun rose on China, Hudson Taylor was worshipping God. In other words, the rising sun of China never saw Hudson Taylor not worshipping the Lord for fifty-one years. This is how Hudson Taylor cultivated the intimacy and relationship with the Lord daily. It was the secret of his ministry.

Prayer

Dear Jesus, I know I cannot do anything apart from You. I need You. I want to be connected with You closely, fully, and wholly. Help me to remain in You every single day of my life, that we may bring forth fruit and fruit that will remain.

Two Ways of Life

One of the most beautiful characteristics of the Bible is its transparency. We can see its personages, patriarchs, prophets, kings, apostles, and all their heroes described as they are without covering up and without hiding their fears, mistakes, shame, failures, and weaknesses. The Word of God is teaching us how precious it is to live in the light, because

> God is light; in him there is no darkness at all. If we claim to have fellowship with him and yet walk in the darkness, we lie and do not live out the truth. But if we walk in the light, as he is in the light, we have fellowship with one another, and the blood of Jesus, his Son, purifies us from all sin. (1 John 1:5–7)

It may be hard and humbling, but is in the light that we find forgiveness, deliverance, freedom, reconciliation, fellowship, and peace with God and one another.

The book of Psalms, in Hebrew is called *Tehilim* or praises, and it means poems to be sung with stringed instruments, is the playlist of songs of the Hebrews in the old times, *but also is Tefilot*, or a collection of prayers where the authors open up their hearts, exposing themselves as they are before the holy God[23]. It is noteworthy that many times the psalmist brought his fears, worries, sufferings, and questions to God with anguish in his heart but finished with praises of joy.

The experience and the message of the Psalms are: come to God with whatever difficulty you may have, come to the light, and open your heart to Him. You will find that He is your defender, your shield, your fortress, and the Rock of your salvation.

The book of Psalms is one of the most cherished books ever written because it is real-life experience. It has brought so much comfort, healing, and encouragement for people of all ages in the whole world for the last three thousand years. We will study the first Psalm.

> Blessed is the one who does not walk in step with the wicked or stand in the way that sinners take or sit in the company of mockers, but whose delight is in the law of the LORD, and who meditates on his law day and night. That person is like a tree planted by streams of water, which yields its fruit in season and whose leaf does not wither—whatever they do prospers. Not so the wicked! They are like chaff that the wind blows away. Therefore the wicked will not stand in the judgment, nor sinners in the assembly of the righteous. For the LORD watches over the way of the righteous, but the way of the wicked leads to destruction.

---

[23] Tyndale, New Bible Dictionary, Inter-vasity Press, Tyndale House Publishers, Wheaton IL, 1962

Psalm 1 is a didactic Psalm and teaches us that the whole of humanity can be divided in two groups that follows two different ways of life: the righteous and the wicked. How can we know which is the path we are walking in? We need to ask ourselves three questions.

1. *Where is our delight?*

We can see that the way of the unrighteous is a downward progression: walk with the wicked, stand with sinners, and sit with the mockers. The unrighteous start with a careless curiosity, walking in step with the wicked. They just allow their eyes to see what is going on up there, and then they stop and stand in the way that sinners take. They become interested and enjoy what they offer for a while, and soon they are sitting in the company of mockers. They are part of the group, entangled, ensnared, and entrapped with those who openly live in sin. They cannot escape anymore.

The righteous, on the other hand, avoid the possibility or the appearance of evil. The righteous know there is danger in some places. They wisely avoid situations where they may fall in sin.

Do you remember what happened to Joseph in the Bible? He was a well-built, handsome, and young single man in a foreign country. Joseph's master's wife took notice of Joseph and said, "Come to bed with me!" What was his reply? "How could I do such a wicked thing and sin against God?" And though she spoke to Joseph day after day, he refused to go to bed with her or even be with her. One day he went into the house to attend to his duties, and none of the household servants was inside. She caught him by his cloak and said, "Come to bed with me!" But he left his cloak in her hand and ran out of the house. He ran because he knew the danger of falling into sin. The best way to avoid sin is to be far away from situations where you may fall in it and to be closer to God.

Should we cut all communication with the unrighteous? Not at all. The righteous do not love the world in the sense of lust or desiring it for themselves. They do love in the sense that they want it in the light, in righteousness, and in the kingdom of God. The righteous are not part of the world, but they are actively engaged in it. They are like ambassadors of another country. They are here to serve, to represent and bring a message of love and hope from their King. Jesus said you are the light of the world.

If the delight of the righteous is not in the ways of sinners, where is it? The delight of the righteous is in the law of the Lord. This is their love, pleasure, and passion. The highlight of their day is the time spent alone with the Word of God. "His word is a lamp for his feet, a light on his path" (Ps. 119:105). This is the manual where the righteous learn how to be loving husbands, godly wives, wise fathers, caring mothers, and trustworthy professionals. The Word of God transforms the righteous person's mind-set, breaks his pride, heals his wounds, and comforts his heart because it is alive and active, sharper than any double-edged sword. It penetrates even to dividing of soul and spirit, joints and marrow. It judges the thoughts and attitudes of the heart (Heb. 4:12). The Word of God gives us a precise diagnosis of our spiritual condition and convicts us of sin. It changes us.

In Brazil many years ago there was a famous robber called Benedito de Lima César, known as seven fingers. His phenomenal escapes from the most secure prisons in the country would make an exciting movie in Hollywood, but one day he was put in jail in a city called Bauru. Somebody there gave him a Bible, and he instantly threw it to the wall. The next day he found the Bible opened on the floor, and the light from outside was shining on in its pages. He was captivated by this heavenly vision and started to read the book. His heart was broken, and he confessed his sins. He found forgiveness and the warm embrace of the Father. Joy and peace filled his heart. He was a new man. He started to humbly serve others, and not long after he received conditional freedom. He went out to visit prisons and hospitals, telling the wonders of the love of God. He was transformed by reading the Word, "Because it is the power of God that brings salvation to everyone who believes" (Rom. 1:16). Do you want to be transformed? Do you want to change? Read it. But it must not be a quick, superficial reading.

Meditate in the Word of God day and night. To meditate implies to take time, thinking, asking, enquiring, learning, memorizing, chewing, absorbing, and digesting. Technology is evolving all the time. This information may sound like archeology for some of you, but I read in the newspaper a long time ago an article about astronomy that I thought was very interesting. It was about an astronomical observatory that could detect more stars than any other at that time. It was built with photographic film that is exposed to the light of the universe for many, many hours, so it was able to detect the farthest stars that others could not. In the same way, we need to expose our minds to the Word of God. Time. How much time do you spend in the Word of God? It is not a snapshot photo. It is not a quick glimpse. Meditation is a gaze, a long exposure of our minds to the light of Scripture until all the cells of our brain are impressed with the Word of the living God. Where is your delight? Blessed is the one whose delight is in the law of the Lord and who meditates on His law day and night. God have the same prescription for blessing and success to Joshua.

> After the death of Moses the servant of the LORD, the LORD said to Joshua son of Nun, Moses' aide: "Moses my servant is dead. Now then, you and all these people, get ready to cross the Jordan River into the land I am about to give to them—to the Israelites. I will give you every place where you set your foot, as I promised Moses. Your territory will extend from the desert to Lebanon, and from the great river, the Euphrates—all the Hittite country—to the Mediterranean Sea in the west. No one will be able to stand against you all the days of your life. As I was with Moses, so I will be with you; I will never leave you nor forsake you. Be strong and courageous, because you will lead these people to inherit the land I swore to their ancestors to give them.

> "Be strong and very courageous. Be careful to obey all the law my servant Moses gave you; do not turn from it to the right or to the left, that you may be successful wherever you go. Keep this Book of the Law always on your lips; meditate on it day and night, so that you

may be careful to do everything written in it. Then you will be prosperous and successful. Have I not commanded you? Be strong and courageous. Do not be afraid; do not be discouraged, for the LORD your God will be with you wherever you go. (Josh. 1:1–9)

As human beings, it is very easy for us to be afraid or discouraged, to be anxious or depressed. God gives us a word of encouragement: "Be strong and courageous. Do not be afraid. Do not be discouraged, for I am with you always wherever you go. I will never leave you nor forsake you." He is the only perfect person in the universe who will never disappoint you. He is the only invincible, unchangeable Savior who we can trust all the time. If the almighty God is with you, why should you be afraid? If the Everlasting Father said, "I will never leave you nor forsake you," why should you be discouraged? But also God gives us the following three commands to be successful:

1. Meditate in the book of the law day and night.
2. Be careful to obey all the law and do everything written in it.
3. Keep this book of the law always on your lips.

Meditate day and night, obey it all, and never stop talking about it. Meditate, obey, and talk. Talk to your children, talk to your friends, and talk to your neighbor.

> For as the rain and the snow come down from heaven,
> And do not return there without watering the earth
> And making it bear and sprout, And furnishing seed

to the sower and bread to the eater; So will My word
be which goes forth from My mouth; It will not return
to Me empty, Without accomplishing what I desire,
And without succeeding in the matter for which I sent
it. (Isa. 55:10–11)

In the same way the water comes from above and gives life
to the earth, so the Word that comes from God gives life to the
world. Share the Word of God all the time. It will give light,
hope, and life. It will change your family, your company, and
your community. The Word of God is simply the power to change
the world.

The second question we need to ask ourselves is:

2. *Where is our dependency? Where is our trust, our security?
    Are we relying in our own intelligence, strength, paycheck,
    or bank account?*

The difference between the righteous and the wicked is not
fundamentally in their deeds but in their foundation. The wicked
are also called ungodly. These people became wicked because they
chose to live apart from God, an ungodly life, as if God didn't
exist. They are empty, without life, because they refused to trust in
God and chose to chase after the wind of this world. The wicked
are compared to chaff, like husks of wheat or other cereal. It was
separated from the grain by threshing, whereupon it usually blew
away because it was lighter than the grain. The wicked are frequently
likened to chaff in Scripture because there is no content in it. It is
empty, useless. They will disappear as chaff is blown away.

The righteous are not righteous by their own virtue but because they stuck to the ground and stretched their roots, looking for the truth of the real meaning of life, and found the fountain of life in God. He chose to trust in God, to be connected, grounded, rooted, established, and based in his love, so he became a tree, strong, resilient, and fruitful, even in times of drought because its roots are connected with the streams of living waters, the source of all life, strength, and love that is God Himself and His Word that endures forever. His righteousness is a gift from God.

In the spring, we see the powerful process of life before our eyes. Seemingly dead trees start to sprout after the winter. Small green leaves grow day by day on new branches and bud into beautiful flowers. In a short time, we see an explosion of life all over. They grow, they blossom, and they bear fruit because they have life. The righteous are compared to a tree planted by streams of water, which yields its fruit in season and whose leaf does not wither, a symbol of permanence or long life. Whatever they do prospers.

That is why Jesus taught:

> Therefore everyone who hears these words of mine and puts them into practice is like a wise man who built his house on the rock. The rain came down, the streams rose, and the winds blew and beat against that house; yet it did not fall, because it had its foundation on the rock. But everyone who hears these words of mine and does not put them into practice is like a foolish man who built his house on sand. The rain came down, the streams rose, and the winds blew and

beat against that house, and it fell with a great crash.
(Matt. 7:24–27)

Dear friends, everything in this world, economies, politics, polices, empires and companies change, our own thoughts and emotions change, they pass away as the wind. The only stable, immovable, trustworthy, eternal foundation in the universe is the almighty God and His word. Is He your delight and dependency?

If our delight and dependency are settled, so is ...

3. Our destiny

> Therefore the wicked will not stand in the judgment,
> nor sinners in the assembly of the righteous. For the
> LORD watches over the way of the righteous, but the
> way of the wicked leads to destruction. (Ps. 1:5–6)

As Matthew Henry said, "The punishment of the wicked is compared to threshing and their end will be like chaff which is burned. Those that by their own sin and folly make themselves as chaff will be found so before the whirlwind and fire of divine wrath[24]. The destiny of the wicked is sealed by their own choice. Because they refused the love of God, they went astray from the shepherd, rejected the fountain of living waters, they became dried, dead, empty chaff blown by the wind to the fire of destruction.

> How blessed is the man who fears the Lord, who greatly
> delights in His commandments. His descendants will

---

[24]   Matthew Henry Commentary, http://www.biblegateway.com

be mighty on earth; the generation of the upright will
be blessed. (Ps. 112:1–2)

Never has this been more graphically illustrated than in the
life of Jonathan Edwards (born in 1703, pastor, theologian, and
president of what became the Princeton University). He was a
man wholly devoted to Jesus Christ. At age seventeen, he married
Sarah Pierpont. On their wedding night, they committed their
marriage to the Lord. By 1900, their descendants included three
hundred pastors, missionaries, and theologians; one hundred
attorneys, sixty judges (one dean of a law school); sixty doctors
(one dean of a medical school); sixty authors of fine classics; one
hundred professors and fourteen presidents of universities; three
mayors of large cities; three state governors; a controller of the US
Treasury; and a vice president of America who became president,
Theodore Roosevelt. What a tremendous impact on their country
and the world in literature, law, science, and all of society a young
couple can make just because one day they decided to submit their
lives to Jesus Christ.

Another man who lived in the same time was Max Dukes
(born in 1700). He was an unbeliever who married an unsaved
woman. They neither honored God nor lived principled lives.
Among their twelve hundred known descendants in 1900: 310
were professional vagrants; 440 wrecked their lives by wild living;
130 went to jail (seven for murder, on average for thirteen years);
over one hundred became alcoholics; sixty were habitual thieves;
and 190 were prostitutes. Twenty became tradesmen (ten of whom
learned their trade in jail). The researcher who compiled these

statistics estimated that Max Dukes's descendants cost the state of New York $1.5 million.[25]

I remember a story I heard in Sunday school one day and never forgot. There is a place in the Andes where if a raindrop falls in one side of a tree, it will end up in the Atlantic Ocean, but if it falls just one millimeter to the other side, it will end up in the Pacific Ocean. In the beginning, it is just a few millimeters apart, but at the end, it will be thousands of kilometers away. There is a saying that was published anonymously in 1881 by the Unitarian Sunday School Society that says, "Sow a thought, and you reap an act. Sow an act, and you reap a habit. Sow a habit, and you reap a character. Sow a character, and you reap a destiny."

Neither Jonathan Edwards nor Max Dukes could imagine what their descendants would be like two hundred years later. But each small decision they made impacted the future destiny of generations to come. In the same way, each small decision we make today will impact the future of our descendants not only in two hundred years but also throughout all eternity.

We should not think, though, that success before men is the same as success before God. The currency of this world is worth nothing in heaven. The rules and values in heaven are quite different from on earth. Mother Theresa of Calcutta (1910–1997) once said, "It's not about how much you do, but how much love you put into what you do that counts." That is why Jesus said: "But many who are first will be last, and many who are last will be first" (Matt. 19:30).

---

[25] http://www.joymag.co.za/article.php?id=96.

I would like to finish by telling you about Charles Studd (1860–1931). When he was young, he had wealth and fame as the captain of a cricket team in England, but he counted it as loss and came to Shanghai in 1885 as a missionary. (Seven from Cambridge came to China with him). At that time, there were no subways, buses, or taxis, so he would walk thousands of kilometers, visiting the villages sharing the Word of God. In those days there was no shoes of his size in China, so his feet were bleeding most of the time. After many years in this country, in1900 he was called and went to share the gospel in India. In 1908, he saw a plaque with the words: "Cannibals want missionaries" (this was an invitation to mission in Africa). He went to Africa in 1910, where he served till the end of his life.

Humanly speaking, this does not seem like a successful life at all. But from the perspective of God, what matters is not how much you have or how much you do but how much you love—not in words but in acts. How many thousands of people in China and India and Africa were blessed by his life of obedience. At the age of fifty-two, when he decided to go to Africa and people started to ask why, his reply was, "If Jesus Christ is God and died for me, then no sacrifice can be too great for me to make for Him."

The righteous are blessed, and whatever they do prospers. Do you want to be blessed and prosperous from the perspective of heaven? It doesn't matter what your past looks like; you have a choice before you today. Choose now to turn away from the ways of the wicked. Find your delight in the Word of God and your dependency in God Himself, and your destiny will be blessed and successful indeed.

Prayer

Dear Father, I know there are things that are not right in my life. I want to turn away from them. Forgive me. I want to surrender my life to You.

Personal Testimony:

At sixteen years of age I perceived the feebleness and transience of life, how it could just pass away all of a sudden, and how I was unprepared, in need of security and meaning. Soon after that I was introduced to the Bible by missionaries that came to our town in Brazil and found in Jesus forgiveness, assurance, love, a new life, and purpose. At that time I gave my life to Him, and my desire since then is to follow Him wherever He leads.

I cannot forget the message a patient who was going through a very difficult situation and divorce sent me one day, "Can you mend a broken heart?" I was not able to answer that day, but this question made me think for a long time: What can we do as health professionals? How complex is human nature, how can we help families in this city?

I would like to say now: I cannot mend a broken heart, but I know a Person that can. He is the One that said:

"The Spirit of the Lord God is upon Me, Because the Lord has anointed Me To preach good tidings to the poor; He has sent Me to heal the brokenhearted, To proclaim liberty to the captives, And the opening of the prison to those who are bound;"(Isaiah 61:1 NKJV). His name is Jesus.

Would you like to know Him?

The author can be contacted at: <u>lincoln.miyasaka@gmail.com</u>